70 Colon Cancer Juice and Meal Recipes:

Enrich Your Nutrition the Natural Way to Prevent and Fight Cancer

By

Joe Correa CSN

COPYRIGHT

This publication is designed to provide accurate and authoritative information in regard to the subject matter covered. It is sold with the understanding that neither the author nor the publisher is engaged in rendering medical advice. If medical advice or assistance is needed, consult with a doctor. This book is considered a guide and should not be used in any way detrimental to your health. Consult with a physician before starting this nutritional plan to make sure it's right for you.

ACKNOWLEDGEMENTS

This book is dedicated to my friends and family that have had mild or serious illnesses so that you may find a solution and make the necessary changes in your life.

70 Colon Cancer Juice and Meal Recipes:

Enrich Your Nutrition the Natural Way to Prevent and Fight Cancer

By

Joe Correa CSN

CONTENTS

ABOUT THE AUTHOR

After years of Research, I honestly believe in the positive effects that proper nutrition can have over the body and mind. My knowledge and experience has helped me live healthier throughout the years and which I have shared with family and friends. The more you know about eating and drinking healthier, the sooner you will want to change your life and eating habits.

Nutrition is a key part in the process of being healthy and living longer so get started today. The first step is the most important and the most significant.

INTRODUCTION

70 Colon Cancer Juice and Meal Recipes: Enrich Your Nutrition the Natural Way to Prevent and Fight Cancer

By Joe Correa CSN

Colon cancer is a common disease which happens when tumorous growths develop in the large intestine. This serious disease is the third most common cause of cancer-related deaths in the United States which is why recognizing the symptoms and changing some lifestyle habits can be a lifesaver.

The most common symptoms you definitely have to keep in check are:

- A sudden change in your bowel movements
- Any type of rectal bleeding is a potential colon cancer symptom
- Intense abdominal pain
- Frequent weakness or fatigue
- Sudden and unexplained weight loss

However, you have to keep in mind that most people don't experience any of these symptoms in the early stages of the disease. This is why a regular physical exam is very important if for some reason you suspect abnormalities.

Another important step you have to take in order to prevent this terrible and extremely dangerous disease is definitely a dietary lifestyle change. This life-saving decision will permanently change the way you eat, and most importantly, a healthy diet will change the way your digestive tract handles food. This means that with just a couple of simple steps, your body will start to change and you will feel much better. You will have to change the way you eat and adopt some long-term diet habits. Only this will permanently clean your digestive tract and reduce the risk of colon cancer.

But, I have to point out that in order to be 100% sure you're healthy, the diet, by itself, won't be enough. A healthy diet combined with regular exercise is the only way to successfully fight off this disease.

This beautiful collection of colon cancer preventing juice recipes will become your guide in leading a healthy life. These juices are full of fibers that will clean your entire digestive tract and wash away all the toxins you've been collecting over the years. But, that's not all, these juices were carefully chosen to fully satisfy your taste and make you want more! They are amazingly simple to prepare. Within just a couple of minutes you will have a glass full of nutrients your body needs on a daily basis.

Make sure to try them all and I wish you the best luck in your journey back to health!

70 COLON CANCER JUICE AND MEAL RECIPES: ENRICH YOUR NUTRITION THE NATURAL WAY TO PREVENT AND FIGHT CANCER

JUICES

1.   Apple Ginger Juice

Ingredients:

1 large Granny Smith's apple, cored

½ cup of collard greens

1 tsp of ginger, ground

1 large cucumber

¼ cup of fresh parsley

Preparation:

Wash the apple and cut lengthwise in half. Remove the core and chop into small pieces. Set aside.

Wash the collard greens thoroughly under cold running water using a large colander. Drain and torn into small pieces. Set aside.

Wash the cucumber and cut into thin slices. Set aside.

Rinse the parsley and chop into small pieces. Set aside.

Now, combine apple, collard greens, cucumber, and parsley in a juicer and process until juiced. trans

Transfer to serving glasses and add few ice cubes.

Serve immediately.

Nutritional information per serving: Kcal: 96, Protein: 3.1g, Carbs: 28.7g, Fats: 1.2g

2.   Carrot Turnip Juice

Ingredients:

2 large carrots, sliced

1 cup of turnip greens, torn

1 cup of cauliflower, chopped

1 large radish, chopped

¼ tsp of ginger, ground

2 oz of water

Preparation:

Wash and peel the carrots. Cut into thin slices and set aside.

Wash the turnip greens thoroughly under cold running water. Drain and torn into small pieces. Set aside.

Trim off the outer leaves of the cauliflower. Wash it and chop into small pieces. Fill the measuring cup and reserve the rest for later.

Wash the radish and chop into small pieces. Set aside.

Wash the radish and chop into small pieces. Set aside.

Now, combine cauliflower, carrots, radish, and turnip greens in a juicer and process until juiced. Transfer to a serving glass and stir in the ginger and water.

Add some ice and serve immediately.

Nutritional information per serving: Kcal: 75, Protein: 4.3g, Carbs: 23.3g, Fats: 0.8g

3.   Lemon Grapefruit Juice

Ingredients:

2 whole lemons, peeled and halved

1 whole grapefruit, peeled and wedged

1 cup of mango, chunked

1 small Granny Smith's apple, cored

¼ tsp of ginger, ground

Preparation:

Peel the lemons and cut each lengthwise in half. Set aside.

Peel the grapefruit and divide into wedges. Cut each wedge in half and set aside.

Peel the mango and cut into chunks. Fill the measuring cup and reserve the rest for later. Set aside.

Wash the apple and cut lengthwise in half. Remove the core and cut into bite-sized pieces. Set aside.

Now, combine lemon, mango, grapefruit, and apple in a juicer and process until juiced. Transfer to a serving glass and stir in the ginger.

Add few ice cubes and serve immediately.

Enjoy!

Nutritional information per serving: Kcal: 65, Protein: 4.5g, Carbs: 16.8g, Fats: 0.8g

4.   Apple Celery Juice

Ingredients:

1 small Golden Delicious apple, cored

1 cup of celery, chopped

1 cup of apricots, chopped

1 cup of strawberries, chopped

¼ tsp of cinnamon, ground

Preparation:

Wash the apple and cut lengthwise in half. Remove the core and cut into small pieces. Set aside.

Wash the celery and chop into small pieces. Set aside.

Wash the apricots and cut in half. Remove the pits and chop into small pieces. Fill the measuring cup and reserve the rest for later. Set aside.

Wash the strawberries and remove the stems. Cut into small pieces and fill the measuring cup. Reserve the rest for later.

Now, combine apple,celery, apricots, and strawberries in a juicer and process until juiced. Transfer to a serving glass and stir in the cinnamon.

Add some ice and serve immediately.

Nutritional information per serving: Kcal: 170, Protein: 4.3g, Carbs: 49.9g, Fats: 1.4g

5.   Broccoli Lime Juice

Ingredients:

2 cups of broccoli, chopped

1 whole lime, peeled and halved

2 cups of kale, chopped

1 cup of cucumber, sliced

1 whole lemon, peeled and halved

1 oz of water

Preparation:

Wash the broccoli and trim off the outer leaves. Cut into small pieces and fill the measuring cup. Reserve the rest in the refrigerator.

Peel the lime and lemon. Cut each fruit lengthwise in half and set aside.

Wash the kale thoroughly under cold running water. Drain and chop into small pieces. Set aside.

Wash the cucumber and cut into thin slices. Fill the measuring cup and reserve the rest for later.

Now, combine broccoli, kale, cucumber, lime, and lemon in a juicer and process until juiced. Transfer to a serving glass and stir in the water.

Sprinkle with some mint for some extra taste, but it's optional.

Refrigerate for 10 minutes before serving.

Enjoy!

Nutritional information per serving: Kcal: 116, Protein: 12.1g, Carbs: 34.8g, Fats: 2.2g

6.   Lemon Pineapple Juice

Ingredients:

1 whole lemon, peeled

1 cup of black grapes

1 cup of pineapple, chunked

1 whole grapefruit, peeled and wedged

¼ tsp of cinnamon, ground

Preparation:

Peel the lemon and cut lengthwise in half. Set aside.

Using a sharp paring knife, cut the top of the pineapple. Gently remove all hard skin and cut into chunks. Fill the measuring cup and reserve the in the refrigerator.

Rinse the grapes thoroughly under cold running water. Remove the stems and fill the measuring cup. Set aside.

Peel the grapefruit and divide into wedges. Cut each wedge in half and set aside.

Now, combine lemon,grapes, pineapple, and grapefruit in a juicer and process until juiced. Transfer to a serving glass and stir in the cinnamon.

Add some crushed ice and serve immediately.

Nutritional information per serving: Kcal: 230, Protein: 4g, Carbs: 69.1g, Fats: 1.1g

7.   Pepper Lettuce Juice

Ingredients:

1 large yellow bell pepper, chopped

1 cup of Romaine lettuce, chopped

1 cup of fennel, sliced

1 cup of cucumber, sliced

1 small zucchini, cubed

Preparation:

Wash the bell pepper and cut lengthwise in half. Remove the stem and seeds. Cut into small pieces and set aside.

Wash the Romaine lettuce thoroughly under cold running water. Drain and chop into small pieces. Set aside.

Trim off the fennel bulb and remove the green parts. Wash it and cut into small pieces. Fill the measuring cup and reserve the rest for later. Set aside.

Wash the cucumber and cut into thin slices. Fill the measuring cup and reserve the rest for later.

Wash the zucchini and cut into small cubes. Set aside.

Now, combine bell pepper, lettuce,fennel, cucumber, and zucchini in a juicer and process until juiced. Transfer to a serving glass and refrigerate for 5 minutes before serving.

Nutritional information per serving: Kcal: 85, Protein: 5.3g, Carbs: 25.2g, Fats: 1.1g

8.   Cantaloupe Pear Juice

Ingredients:

1 cup of cantaloupe, peeled and chopped

1 medium-sized pear, chopped

1 whole leek, chopped

1 whole lime, peeled

1 oz of coconut water

¼ tsp of ginger, ground

Preparation:

Cut the cantaloupe in half. Scoop out the seeds and flesh. Cut and peel one large wedge. Chop into chunks and fill the measuring cup. Reserve the rest of the cantaloupe in a refrigerator.

Wash the pear lengthwise in half. Remove the core and cut into bite-sized pieces. Set aside.

Wash the leek thoroughly under cold running water. Drain and chop into small pieces. Set aside.

Peel the lime and cut lengthwise in half. Set aside.

Now, combine cantaloupe, pear, leek, and lime in a juicer and process until juiced. Transfer to a serving glass and stir in the coconut water and ginger.

Add some ice, or refrigerate for 5 minutes before serving.

Nutritional information per serving: Kcal: 184, Protein: 3.5g, Carbs: 56.2g, Fats: 0.8g

9. Radish Brussels Sprout Juice

Ingredients:

2 large radishes, chopped

2 cups of Brussels sprouts, halved

1 small zucchini, chopped

1 cup of cucumber, sliced

2 large carrots, sliced

¼ tsp of turmeric, ground

Preparation:

Wash the radishes and trim off the green parts. Slightly peel and cut into small pieces. Set aside.

Wash the Brussels sprouts and trim off the outer layers. Cut into halves and fill the measuring cups. Reserve the rest in the refrigerator.

Wash the zucchini and cut into thin slices. Set aside.

Wash the cucumber and cut into thin slices. Fill the measuring cup and reserve the rest for later.

Wash and peel the carrots. Cut into thin slices and set aside.

Now, combine radishes, Brussels sprouts, zucchini, cucumber, and carrots in a juicer and process until juiced. Transfer to a serving glass and stir in the turmeric. Refrigerate for 15 minutes before serving.

Nutritional information per serving: Kcal: 118, Protein: 9.2g, Carbs: 35.7g, Fats: 1.3g

10.   Swiss Chard Lime Juice

Ingredients:

½ cup of Swiss chard

1 large lime, peeled

½ cup of fresh basil

2 large green apples, cored

¼ cup of fresh mint

Preparation:

Wash the Swiss chard and basil thoroughly and roughly chop it. Set aside.

Peel the lime and cut into quarters. Set aside.

Wash the mint leaves and soak in water for 10 minutes. Set aside.

Wash the apples and remove the core. Cut into bite-sized pieces and set aside.

Now combine, Swiss chard, lime, basil, and apples, and mint in a juicer. Process until juiced. Transfer to serving glasses and add some ice before serving.

Garnish with some extra mint leaves and add some ice before serving.

Enjoy!

Nutritional information per serving: Kcal: 114, Protein: 2.3g, Carbs: 30.4g, Fats: 0.2g

11. Pomegranate Apple Juice

Ingredients:

½ cup of pomegranate seeds

1 large green apple, cored

½ cup of fresh kale

¼ tsp of ginger, ground

3-4 fresh mint leaves

Preparation:

Cut the top of the pomegranate fruit using a sharp knife. slice down to each of the white membranes inside of the fruit. Pop the seeds into a medium sized bowl.

Wash the apple and remove the core. Cut into bite-sized pieces and set aside.

Wash thoroughly the kale. Drain and roughly chop it. Set aside.

Process the pomegranate seeds, apple, and kale in a juicer until well juiced.

Transfer to serving glasses and stir in the ginger. Add some water to adjust the thickness and garnish with mint leaves.

Add few ice cubes and serve immediately.

Nutritional information per serving: Kcal: 143, Protein: 6.2g, Carbs: 41.2g, Fats: 2.4g

12.   Cucumber Pineapple Juice

Ingredients:

1 large cucumber

1 cup of pineapple, chopped

3 celery stalks

½ cup of fresh spinach

¼ tsp of ginger, ground

Preparation:

Wash and slice the cucumber into thick slices. Set aside.

Peel the pineapple and cut into chunks. Set aside.

Combine celery and spinach in a colander and wash under cold running water. Roughly chop the spinach and celery.

Combine cucumber, pineapple, celery, and spinach in a juicer and process until well juiced.

Transfer to serving glasses and stir in the ginger. Add a pinch of turmeric for some extra flavor. However, it's optional.

Serve immediately.

Nutritional information per serving: Kcal: 109, Protein: 3.3g, Carbs: 61.2g, Fats: 1.3g

13.   Broccoli Carrot Juice

Ingredients:

1 cup of fresh broccoli

4 large carrots

2 cups of cauliflower, chopped

1 large green apple, cored

1 small ginger root slice, 1-inch

Preparation:

Wash the broccoli and chop it into small pieces.

Wash the carrots and cut into small pieces.

Wash the apple and remove the core. Cut into bite-sized pieces and set aside.

Wash the cauliflower under cold running water, and place it in a medium-sized bowl. Chop into small pieces and add water enough to cover it. Set aside to soak for 15 minutes.

Peel the ginger root and cut into halves.

Now, process cauliflower, broccoli, apple, carrot, and ginger root. Transfer to serving glasses and add some ice cubes before serving.

Enjoy!

Nutritional information per serving: Kcal: 136, Protein: 6.3g, Carbs: 42.8g, Fats: 1.2g

14.   Sweet Potato Peach Juice

Ingredients:

2 medium-sized sweet potatoes, pre-cooked

1 large peach, pitted and halved

¼ tsp of ginger, ground

¼ tsp of cinnamon, ground

Preparation:

Peel the potatoes and place them in a pot of boiling water. Cook until fork-tender. Remove from the heat and drain well. Cut the potatoes into small pieces and set aside to cool completely.

Wash the peach and cut into halves. Remove the pit and chop into bite-sized pieces. Set aside.

Now, combine potatoes and peach in a juicer and process until juiced. Transfer to serving glasses and stir in the ginger and cinnamon.

Add some ice and serve immediately.

Nutritional information per serving: Kcal: 159, Protein: 5.2g, Carbs: 50.1g, Fats: 0.9g

15. Bok Choy Apple Juice

Ingredients:

1 small baby bok choy

1 large green apple, cored

¼ cup of fresh basil

1 medium-sized leek

2 large carrots

4-5 fresh kale leaves

Preparation:

Discard the ends of the bokchoy stems. Wash it thoroughly and chop it into small pieces. Set aside.

Wash the apple and remove the core. Cut into bite-sized pieces and set aside.

Wash the leek and chop into small pieces. set aside.

Combine basil and kale in a colander and wash under cold running water. Chop roughly with your hands. Set aside.

Wash the carrots and chop into thick slices. Set aside.

Now, process all prepared ingredients in a juicer. Transfer to serving glasses and refrigerate for 10 minutes before serving.

Enjoy!

Nutritional information per serving: Kcal: 169, Protein: 2.3g, Carbs: 46.2g, Fats: 1.9g

16.   Cantaloupe Lettuce Juice

Ingredients:

1 cup of cantaloupe, peeled

1 small Romaine lettuce head

1 tbsp of coconut, grated

½ cup of fresh basil

1 large cucumber

Preparation:

Peel the cantaloupe and cut into chunks. Reserve the rest of the cantaloupe in the refrigerator.

Wash the lettuce thoroughly. Roughly chop with hands and set aside.

Wash the cucumber and cut into thick slices. Set aside.

Wash the basil and chop with hands. Set aside.

Now, combine cantaloupe, lettuce, basil, and cucumber in a juicer and process until juiced.

Transfer to serving glasses and stir in the coconut. You can add some liquid honey for some extra taste, but this is optional.

Refrigerate for 15 minutes before serving.

Nutritional information per serving: Kcal: 112, Protein: 2.3g, Carbs: 22.6g, Fats: 1.1g

17.   Mediterranean Citrus Juice

Ingredients:

½ tsp of fresh rosemary

3 large grapefruits, peeled

3 large oranges, peeled

1 whole lemon, peeled

Preparation:

Wash the grapefruits and cut into bite-sized pieces. Set aside.

Peel the oranges and divide into wedges. Set aside.

Peel the lemon and cut into quarters. Process in a juicer until well juiced.

Now, process grapefruits and oranges. Transfer to serving glasses and sprinkle with fresh rosemary for some extra flavor.

If you don't like rosemary, you can replace it with fresh mint.

Add some ice cubes and serve immediately.

Enjoy!

Nutritional information per serving: Kcal: 140, Protein: 3.4g, Carbs: 37.6g, Fats: 0.1g

18.   Orange Cucumber Juice

Ingredients:

2 large oranges, peeled

1 large cucumber, peeled

1 cup of broccoli

1 large carrot, sliced

Preparation:

Peel the oranges and cut into wedges.

Peel the cucumber and cut into bite-sized pieces and aside.

Wash the broccoli thoroughly. Cut into bite-sized pieces and set aside.

Wash and cut the carrot into thin slices. Process in a juicer until juiced. Now, continue to process broccoli, orange wedges, and cucumber.

Stir well with a spoon and add some ice cubes before serving.

Nutritional information per serving: Kcal: 68, Protein: 2.3g, Carbs: 19.7g, Fats: 0.1g

19.   Fennel Pepper Juice

Ingredients:

1 large fennel bulb, trimmed

2 cups of fresh asparagus, trimmed

1 large green bell pepper, seeded

1 large yellow bell pepper, seeded

1 ginger root slice, 1-inch

2 oz of water

Preparation:

Wash the fennel bulb and trim off the wilted outer layers. Cut into small chunks and set aside.

Wash the bell peppers and cut in half. Remove the seeds and cut into small slices. Set aside.

Wash the asparagus and trim off the woody ends. Cut into 1-inch pieces and set aside.

Peel the ginger root slice and set aside.

Now, combine asparagus, fennel, green and yellow bell pepper, and ginger root in a juicer and process until juiced.

Transfer to serving glasses and stir in the water. Refrigerate for 5 minutes before serving and enjoy!

Nutrition information per serving: Kcal: 143, Protein: 12.1g, Carbs: 47.2g, Fats: 1.5g

20.   Zucchini Lemon Juice

Ingredients:

1 large zucchini, chopped

1 large lemon, peeled

1 cup of pumpkin

1 medium-sized yellow apple, cored

1 medium-sized banana

2 oz of water

Preparation:

Peel the zucchini and cut in half. Scrape out the seeds with a spoon. Cut into chunks and set aside.

Peel the lemon and cut lengthwise in half. Set aside.

Peel the pumpkin and cut in half. Scoop out the seeds using a spoon. Cut one large wedge and peel it. Cut into small chunks and set aside. Reserve the rest for later.

Wash the apple and remove the core. Cut into bite-sized pieces and set aside.

Peel the banana and cut into small chunks. Set aside.

Now, process zucchini, lemon, pumpkin, apple, and banana in a juicer. Transfer to serving glasses and stir in the water.

Add some ice and serve immediately.

Nutrition information per serving: Kcal: 254, Protein: 7.5g, Carbs: 72.9g, Fats: 1.9g

21. Green Celery Juice

Ingredients:

1 cup of celery

1 cup of Swiss chards

1 medium-sized apple, cored

1 cup of collard greens

2 tbsp of fresh parsley

4-5 fresh spinach leaves

2 oz of water

Preparation:

Combine Swiss chards, collard greens, celery, and spinach in a colander. Wash thoroughly under cold running water and drain. Torn with hands and set aside.

Wash the apple and remove the core. Cut into bite-sized pieces and set aside.

Now, combine Swiss chards, celery, apple, collard greens, and spinach in a juicer and process until juiced.

Transfer to serving glasses and stir in the water. Add some ice and garnish with fresh parsley.

Enjoy!

Nutrition information per serving: Kcal: 106, Protein: 4.8g, Carbs: 31.3g, Fats: 1.1g

22.   Broccoli Artichoke Juice

Ingredients:

1 cup of fresh broccoli

1 large artichoke head

1 cup of Brussels sprouts, trimmed

1 large lemon, peeled

1 large cucumber

3 tbsp of fresh parsley

Preparation:

Wash the broccoli and chop into small pieces. set aside.

Using a sharp knife, trim off the outer layers of the artichoke. Wash it and cut into bite-sized pieces. Set aside.

Wash the Brussels sprouts and trim off the outer layers. Cut in half and set aside.

Peel the lemon and cut lengthwise in half. Set aside.

Wash the cucumber and cut into thick slices. Set aside.

Now, process Brussels sprouts, broccoli, artichoke, lemon, and cucumber in a juicer.

Transfer to serving glasses and garnish with fresh parsley. Refrigerate for 10 minutes before serving.

Enjoy!

Nutrition information per serving: Kcal: 140, Protein: 13.8g, Carbs: 48.1g, Fats: 1.4g

23.   Apple Lemon Juice

Ingredients:

2 medium-sized Golden Delicious apples

1 large lemon, peeled

1 large cucumber

3 medium-sized celery stalks

A handful of spinach

2 oz of water

Preparation:

Wash the apples and remove the core. Cut into bite-sized pieces and set aside.

Peel the lemon and cut lengthwise in half. Set aside.

Wash the cucumber and cut into thick slices. Set aside.

Wash the celery stalks and cut into 1-inch pieces. Set aside.

Wash the spinach thoroughly and torn with hands. Set aside.

Now, process apples, lemon, cucumber, celery, and spinach in a juicer. Transfer to serving glasses and stir in the water.

Add some ice and serve.

Nutrition information per serving: Kcal: 224, Protein: 5.2g, Carbs: 65.4g, Fats: 1.5g

24.   Swiss Chard Cucumber Juice

Ingredients:

2 cups of Swiss chard

1 large cucumber

1 cup of fresh parsley, torn

1 small yellow apple, cored

1 small orange, peeled

Preparation:

Combine parsley and Swiss chard in a colander and wash thoroughly under cold running water. Drain and torn with hands. Set aside.

Wash the cucumber and cut into thick slices. Set aside.

Wash the apple and remove the core. Cut into bite-sized pieces and set aside.

Peel the orange and divide into wedges. Set aside.

Now, combine parsley, Swiss chard, cucumber apple, and orange in a juicer and process until juiced. Transfer to serving glasses and add some ice before serving.

Enjoy!

Nutrition information per serving: Kcal: 161, Protein: 6.3g, Carbs: 46.3g, Fats: 1.2g

25. Mint Arugula Juice

Ingredients:

1 cup of fresh mint

1 cup of fresh arugula

1 large carrot

1 large orange, peeled

1 large red bell pepper, seeded

Preparation:

Combine mint and arugula in a colander and wash thoroughly under cold running water. Drain and torn with hands. Set aside.

Wash the carrot and cut into thick slices. Set aside.

Peel the orange and divide into wedges. Set aside.

Wash the bell pepper and cut in half. Remove the seeds and chop into small slices. Set aside.

Now, combine mint, arugula, carrot, orange, and bell pepper in a juicer and process until juiced.

Transfer to serving glasses and stir in the water. You can add a pinch of Himalayan salt, but this is optional.

Add some ice and serve immediately.

Nutrition information per serving: Kcal: 153, Protein: 7.9g, Carbs: 47.3g, Fats: 1.3g

26.   Plum Ginger Juice

Ingredients:

5 large plums, pitted

1 cup of fresh broccoli

1 large cucumber

1 medium-sized apple, cored

¼ tsp of ginger, ground

Preparation:

Wash the plums and cut in half. Remove the pits and set aside.

Wash the broccoli and cut into small pieces. Set aside.

Wash the cucumber and cut into thick slices and set aside.

Wash the apple and remove the core. Cut into bite-sized pieces and set aside.

Now, combine plums, broccoli, cucumber, and apple in a juicer and process until juiced.

Transfer to serving glasses and stir in the ginger. Add few ice cubes before serving.

Enjoy!

Nutrition information per serving: Kcal: 268, Protein: 7.6g, Carbs: 77.4g, Fats: 1.9g

27.   Pomegranate Lime Juice

Ingredients:

1 cup of pomegranate seeds

1 large lime, peeled

1 cup of beets, trimmed and chopped

2 large carrots

1 large cucumber

Preparation:

Cut the top of the pomegranate fruit using a sharp knife. Slice down to each of the white membranes inside of the fruit. Pop the seeds into a measuring cup and set aside.

Peel the lime and cut into lengthwise in half. Set aside.

Wash the beets and trim off the green parts. Cut into bite-sized pieces and fill the measuring cup. Reserve the rest for some other juice.

Wash the carrot and cucumber and cut into thick slices. Set aside.

Now, process pomegranate seeds, lime, beets, carrots and cucumber in a juicer.

Transfer to serving glasses and stir in the water. Add some ice and serve!

Nutrition information per serving: Kcal: 194, Protein: 7.2g, Carbs: 57.7g, Fats: 1.9g

28.   Beet Cauliflower Juice

Ingredients:

3 large beets, trimmed

1 cup of cauliflower, chopped

2 cups of green grapes

1 large lemon, peeled

Preparation:

Wash the beets and trim off the green parts. Cut into bite-sized pieces and set

aside.

Trim off the outer leaves of cauliflower. Wash it and cut into small pieces. Fill the measuring cup and reserve the rest for some other juice. Set aside.

Wash the green grapes under cold running water. Set aside.

Peel the lemon and cut lengthwise in half. Set aside.

Now, process beets, grapes, cauliflower, and lemon in a juicer.

Transfer to serving glasses and add some ice cubes before serving.

Enjoy!

Nutrition information per serving: Kcal: 226, Protein: 7.8g, Carbs: 65.8g, Fats: 1.5g

29.   Orange Carrot Juice

Ingredients:

4 large oranges, peeled

1 cup of carrots, sliced

1 cup of broccoli, chopped

1 cup of Brussels sprouts, chopped

1 cup of turnip greens, chopped

1 tbsp of honey

¼ cup of pure coconut water

Preparation:

Peel the oranges and divide into wedges. Set aside.

Wash the carrots and cut into thick slices. Set aside.

Wash the broccoli and cut into small pieces. Set aside.

Wash the Brussels sprouts and trim off the outer layers. Cut in half and set aside.

Wash the turnip greens thoroughly and torn with hands. Set aside.

Now, combine broccoli, Brussels sprouts, carrots, turnip greens, and oranges in a juicer and process until juiced.

Transfer to serving glasses and stir in the honey and coconut water. Add some ice cubes before serving or refrigerate for 5 minutes.

Enjoy!

Nutrition information per serving: Kcal: 367, Protein: 14.47g, Carbs: 116g, Fats: 1.9g

30.   Blackberry Orange Juice

Ingredients:

1 cup of blackberries, fresh

1 large orange, peeled

2 wedges of watermelon, seeded

½ cup of pure coconut water, unsweetened

1 tbsp of honey, raw

Preparation:

Wash the blackberries under cold running water and set aside.

Peel the orange and divide into wedges. Set aside.

Cut the watermelon lengthwise. Cut two large wedges and peel them. Cut into chunks and remove the seeds. Set aside.

Now, combine watermelon, blackberries, and orange in a juicer and process until juiced.

Transfer to serving glasses and stir the coconut water and honey.

Refrigerate for 5 minutes before serving.

Enjoy!

Nutrition information per serving: Kcal: 264, Protein: 7.2g, Carbs: 78.6g, Fats: 1.7g

31.   Tomato Pepper Juice

Ingredients:

2 large tomatoes, peeled

1 cup of red bell peppers, chopped and seeds removed

4 cups of watercress, torn

4 cups of red leaf lettuce, torn

¼ cup of water

Preparation:

Wash the tomatoes and place them in a bowl. Cut into quarters and reserve the juice while cutting. Set aside.

Wash the bell peppers and cut in half. Remove the seeds and roughly chop it. Fill the measuring cup and reserve the rest for some other juice. Set aside.

Combine watercress and red leaf lettuce in a colander. Wash thoroughly under cold running water and torn with hands. Set aside.

Now, combine tomatoes, bell pepper, watercress, and red leaf lettuce in a juicer and process until juiced.

Transfer to serving glasses and stir in the reserved tomato juice and water.

Refrigerate for 5 minutes before serving.

Enjoy!

Nutrition information per serving: Kcal: 106, Protein: 9.2g, Carbs: 27.4g, Fats: 1.5g

32.   Lemon Zucchini Juice

Ingredients:

1 whole lemon, peeled and halved

1 small zucchini, thinly sliced

1 cup of cauliflower, chopped

1 medium artichoke, chopped

1 small ginger knob, chopped

¼ tsp salt

Preparation:

Peel the lemon and cut lengthwise in half. Set aside.

Wash the zucchini and thinly slice it. Set aside.

Trim off the outer layer of the cauliflower. Cut into bite-sized pieces and wash it. Fill the measuring cup and sprinkle with some salt. Set aside.

Trim off the outer layers of the artichoke using a sharp paring knife. Cut into bite-sized pieces and set aside.

Peel the ginger knob and chop into small pieces. Set aside.

Now, combine lemon, zucchini, cauliflower, artichoke, and

ginger in a juicer. Process until well juiced.

Transfer to a serving glass and refrigerate for 10 minutes before serving.

Enjoy!

Nutrition information per serving: Kcal: 82, Protein: 8.4g, Carbs: 28.9g, Fats: 1.1g

33.   Broccoli Parsley Juice

Ingredients:

2 cups of broccoli, chopped

1 cup of fresh parsley, torn

1 cup of beets, trimmed and chopped

1 cup of celery, chopped

¼ tsp of turmeric, ground

¼ tsp ginger, ground

Preparation:

Wash the broccoli and trim off the outer layers. Chop into small pieces and set aside.

Rinse the parsley under cold running water and slightly drain. Torn with hands into small pieces and set aside.

Wash and peel the beets. Trim off the green ends and chop into bite-sized pieces. Fill the measuring cup and reserve the rest for later.

Wash the celery stalks and chop it into bite-sized pieces. Fill the measuring cup and set aside.

Now, combine broccoli, parsley, beets, and celery in a juicer and process until juiced. Transfer to a serving glass and stir in the turmeric and ginger.

Refrigerate for 5 minutes before serving.

Nutrition information per serving: Kcal: 109, Protein: 9.8g, Carbs: 31.8g, Fats: 1.5g

34.   Banana Blackberry Juice

Ingredients:

1 cup of blackberries

1 large banana, chunked

1 cup of mango, chunked

1 large orange, peeled

¼ tsp of cinnamon, ground

Preparation:

Place the blackberries in a colander and wash under cold running water. Slightly drain and set aside.

Peel the banana and cut into small chunks. Set aside.

Wash the mango and cut into small chunks. Fill the measuring cup and reserve the rest for later.

Peel the orange and divide into wedges. Cut each wedge in half and set aside.

Now, combine mango, blackberries, banana, and orange in a juicer and process until juiced. Transfer to a serving glass and stir in the cinnamon.

Add few ice cubes and serve immediately.

Nutrition information per serving: Kcal: 296, Protein: 6.6g, Carbs: 91.2g, Fats: 2.1g

35.   Lime Blueberry Juice

Ingredients:

1 whole lime, peeled

1 cup of blueberries

1 cup of fresh spinach, chopped

1 medium-sized orange

1 oz coconut water

1 tbsp fresh mint, torn

Preparation:

Peel the lime and cut lengthwise in half. Set aside.

Place the blueberries in a colander and wash under cold running water. Slightly drain and set aside.

Wash the spinach thoroughly and drain. Chop into small pieces and set aside.

Peel the orange and divide into wedges. Cut each wedge in half and set aside.

Now, combine blueberries, spinach, lime, and orange in a juicer and process until well juiced. Transfer to a serving glass and stir in the coconut water.

Sprinkle with some fresh mint and serve.

Enjoy!

Nutrition information per serving: Kcal: 158, Protein: 8.5g, Carbs: 48.1g, Fats: 1.5g

36.   Tomato Basil Juice

Ingredients:

1 cup of cherry tomatoes, halved

1 cup of Swiss chard, torn

1 cup of basil, torn

1 cup of beets, trimmed

¼ tsp of balsamic vinegar

¼ tsp of salt

1 oz of water

Preparation:

Wash the cherry tomatoes and remove the green stems. Cut in half and fill the measuring cup. Reserve the rest in the refrigerator for some other juice.

Combine basil and Swiss chard in a large colander and rinse thoroughly under cold running water. Drain and torn with hands into small pieces. Set aside.

Wash the beets and trim off the green parts. Cut into thin slices and fill the measuring cup. Reserve the rest for later.

Now, combine cherry tomatoes, Swiss chard, basil, and beets in a juicer and process until juiced. Transfer to a serving glass and stir in the vinegar, salt, and water.

Serve immediately.

Nutrition information per serving: Kcal: 72, Protein: 5.1g, Carbs: 21.6g, Fats: 0.7g

37.   Orange Pear Juice

Ingredients:

1 medium-sized orange, peeled

1 medium-sized pear, chopped

1 cup of fennel, chopped

1 whole lemon, peeled

¼ tsp of cinnamon, ground

1 oz of coconut water

Preparation:

Peel the orange and divide into wedges. Cut each wedge in half and set aside.

Wash the pear and cut in half. Remove the core and cut into small pieces. Set aside.

Trim off the outer wilted layers of the fennel. Roughly chop it and fill the measuring cup. Reserve the rest for later.

Peel the lemon and cut lengthwise in half. Set aside.

Now, combine orange, pear, fennel, and lemon in a juicer and process until well juiced. Transfer to a serving glass and stir in the cinnamon and coconut water.

Refrigerate for 10 minutes before serving.

Enjoy!

Nutrition information per serving: Kcal: 156, Protein: 3.6g, Carbs: 54.2g, Fats: 0.7g

38. Carrot Lemon Juice

Ingredients:

1 large carrot, sliced

1 whole lemon, peeled

1 cup of celery, chopped

1 small Granny Smith's apple, cored

¼ tsp ginger, ground

Preparation:

Wash and peel the carrot. Cut into small slices and set aside.

Wash the celery and cut into small pieces. Set aside.

Peel the lemon and cut lengthwise in half. Set aside.

Wash the apple and cut in half. Remove the core and cut into bite-sized pieces. Set aside.

Now, combine carrot, celery, lemon, and apple in a juicer and process until juiced. Transfer to a serving glass and stir in the water and ginger. Refrigerate for 5 minutes.

Serve immediately.

Nutrition information per serving: Kcal: 105, Protein: 2.4g, Carbs: 32.8g, Fats: 0.7g

MEALS

1.   Brown rice breakfast porridge

Brown rice contains a significant amount of fiber and selenium which substantially reduces the risk of colon cancer. It lowers cholesterol levels and contains antioxidant protection.

Ingredients:

1 cup Cooked brown rice

1 cup Low- fat milk

1 Tbsp. Raspberries

1 Tbsp. Raisins

1 Tbsp. Almond

1 tsp. Cinnamon

1 Tbsp. Honey

1 Egg

¼ tsp. Vanilla extract

1 Tbsp. Butter

Preparation:

Combine the brown rice, milk, raspberries, cinnamon, and honey. Bring to boil. Reduce heat and simmer for 20 minutes. Beat the egg and add the vanilla extract. Stir in the egg into the rice a tablespoon at a time. Add the butter. Continue cooking over low heat for 2 minutes to thicken. Remove from heat. Transfer to a serving plate and drizzle with raisins and almonds on top and enjoy!

Serving Size 148 g

Amount per Serving:

Calories 495 Calories from Fat 108

Total Fat 12.0g

Saturated Fat 5.0g

Trans Fat 0.0g

Cholesterol 97mg

Sodium 77mg

Potassium 358mg

Total Carbohydrates 86.9g

Dietary Fiber 4.6g

Sugars 11.8g

Protein 10.9g

Vitamin A 6% • Vitamin C 2% • Calcium 7% •Iron 14%

2.   Fruity smoothie

The American Cancer Society recommends at least five servings of fruits daily to decrease the risk of cancer. In a recent study, berry extracts slowed cancer growth. Strawberry and raspberry extracts particularly have the greatest effect on reducing colon cancer cells.

Ingredients:

1 Frozen banana, sliced

1 Kiwi

2 cups Frozen strawberries

1 cup Raspberries

1 cup Vanilla yogurt

1/2 cup Freshly squeezed orange

3 Tbsp. Honey

Preparation:

Throw in all ingredients in a blender. Blend well and enjoy!

Serving Size 509 g

Amount per Serving:

Calories 362

Calories from Fat 21

Total Fat 2.3g

Saturated Fat 1.3g

Trans Fat 0.0g

Cholesterol 7mg

Sodium 89mg

Potassium 807mg

Total Carbohydrates 79.3g

Dietary Fiber 10.8g

Sugars 61.0g

Protein 9.3g

Vitamin A 5% • Vitamin C 226% • Calcium 30% •Iron 10%

3.   Kale with mushroom and cheese omelet

Regular consumption of cruciferous vegetables such as kale is effective in lowering the risk of cancer. The cancer-protective biochemical, sulforaphane, blocks enzymes that attracts carcinogens to healthy cells. Researchers estimate that eating lots of cruciferous vegetables could lower your risk of breast and colon cancer by 40 percent

Ingredients:

1 cup Kale, stems removed

½ cup Button mushrooms, halved

4 Eggs

1 Tbsp. Low-fat milk

2 tsp. Butter

1/2 cup Cheddar cheese, shredded

1/8 tsp. Salt

Preparation:

In a medium non-stick skillet, cook kale in olive oil for 5 minutes over medium heat, or until kale is wilted. Transfer to a bowl. In another bowl, whisk eggs and milk until well blended. Melt butter in same skillet over medium heat. Add egg mixture and cook for 6 minutes or until almost set.

Top with cheese. Cook until egg mixture is still slightly moist but not completely set. Spoon kale onto the half of the omelet. Season with salt and pepper. Gently fold the omelet in half. Transfer to plate and enjoy!

Serving Size 180 g

Amount per Serving:

Calories 297

Calories from Fat 198

Total Fat 22.0g

Saturated Fat 11.1g

Trans Fat 0.0g

Cholesterol 368mg

Sodium 492mg

Potassium 380mg

Total Carbohydrates 5.6g

Dietary Fiber 0.7g

Sugars 1.5g

Protein 20.0g

Vitamin A 120% • Vitamin C 68% • Calcium 31% •Iron 16%

4.   Veggie burger with kidney beans

A study shows that consumption of beans reduced the incident of colon cancer. Women who ate four or more servings of beans and other legumes weekly lowered their colon cancer risk to one-third. The compound inositol hexaphosphate found in beans is effective in fighting off cancer.

Ingredients:

4 Whole-wheat burger buns

1 can (15.5 oz.) Kidney beans, drained and mashed

1/2 cup Cooked quinoa

2 Tbsp. Red bell pepper, diced

1 Tbsp. Garlic, minced

2 Tbsp. Onion, minced

1 Tbsp. Fresh basil

1 Tbsp. Fresh basil

½ cup Flax seed

½ tsp. Salt

½ tsp. Pepper

1 Tbsp. Olive oil

Preparation:

In a large bowl, combine all ingredients except for olive oil. Mix using your hands to incorporate all ingredients. Form into 4 patties. In a large skillet, over medium heat, fry the patties in olive oil. Cook until both sides of the burgers are brown. Remove from pan and transfer to a whole wheat bun.

Serving Size 197 g

Amount per Serving:

Calories 415

Calories from Fat 169

Total Fat 18.8g

Saturated Fat 2.5g

Trans Fat 0.0g

Cholesterol 0mg

Sodium 596mg

Potassium 737mg

Total Carbohydrates 47.0g

Dietary Fiber 12.7g

Sugars 6.9g

Protein 12.9g

Vitamin A 82% • Vitamin C 388% •Calcium 6% •Iron 60%

5.   Baked salmon

Moderate intake of fatty fish is beneficial in preventing colon cancer because of its polyunsaturated fatty acid content that have anti-inflammation property.

Ingredients:

1 ½ Tbsp. Extra Virgin Oil

4 Boneless salmon fillets, skin on

1 Tbsp. Fresh thyme

Zest of one lemon

½ tsp. Kosher salt

½ tsp. Ground pepper

½ tsp. Lemon juice

Preparation:

Preheat oven to 275F. Grease a small baking tray with oil. Place salmon fillets, skin side down. In a small bowl, mix remaining oil, lemon zest and thyme. Spread mixture on top of salmon fillets. Season with salt and pepper.

Bake salmon until opaque in the center, or for 17 minutes. Drizzle with lemon.

Serving Size 361 g

Amount per Serving:

Calories 476

Calories from Fat 199

Total Fat 22.1g

Saturated Fat 3.2g

Trans Fat 0.0g

Cholesterol 157mg

Sodium 740mg

Potassium 1386mg

Total Carbohydrates 1.2g

Dietary Fiber 0.7g

Protein 69.3g

Vitamin A 7% • Vitamin C 2% • Calcium 15% • Iron 23%

6.   Lean chicken avocado wrap

A diet rich in red meat increases the risk of colon cancer because of its ability to form toxic substances in the gut that promotes cancer. Eating lean meat like chicken greatly reduces risk from colon-cancer.

Ingredients:

4 Whole-wheat tortilla wrap

2 Tbsp. Shallots, thinly sliced

1 Avocado, mashed

¾ cup Cooked chicken, shredded

¾ cup Cheddar cheese, grated

Preparation:

In a bowl, mix chicken, cheese, thyme and avocados. Spread mixture on tortilla wrap. Form a roll. In a skillet, over medium heat, heat olive oil and place all four tortillas. Cook for 2 minutes until burrito is golden brown and cheese is melted.

Serving Size 205 g

Amount per Serving:

Calories 462

Calories from Fat 317

Total Fat 35.2g

Saturated Fat 13.5g

Trans Fat 0.0g

Cholesterol 85mg

Sodium 303mg

Potassium 661mg

Total Carbohydrates 10.9g

Dietary Fiber 6.7g2

Sugars 0.7g

Protein 27.9g

Vitamin A 14% • Vitamin C 18% • Calcium 33% • Iron 8%

7.   Baked turkey

A healthier alternative to consumption of red and processed meat is consumption of lean meat such as turkey. Turkey breast contains less calories and fats than most other cuts of meat. Turkey is rich is selenium which decreases the risk of colorectal cancer.

Ingredients:

1 Tbsp. Onion, coarsely chopped

½ cup Celery, coarsely chopped

½ cup Carrot, coarsely chopped 1

250 g. Turkey fillet

1/8 tsp. Kosher salt

1/8 tsp. Pepper

1/8 tsp. Cayenne pepper

1 tsp. Butter

½ tsp. Fresh rosemary

½ tsp. Fresh sage

Preparation:

Preheat oven to 300F.

In a roasting pan, place onion, celery and carrot. In a small bowl, combine salt, pepper, and cayenne pepper. Rub the salt and pepper mixture on the turkey. Place turkey on top of the vegetables. In a saucepan, over medium heat, melt butter and season with rosemary and sage. Pour melted butter mixture on top of the turkey. Bake turkey uncovered for 45 minutes or until bone is no longer pink and juices run clear. Remove from oven, transfer to a plate and enjoy!

Serving Size 186 g

Amount per Serving:

Calories 249

Calories from Fat 75

Total Fat 8.3g

Saturated Fat 3.3g

Trans Fat 0.0g

Cholesterol 100mg

Sodium 288mg

Potassium 543mg

Total Carbohydrates 4.3g

Dietary Fiber 1.4g

Sugars 1.9g

Protein 37.1g

Vitamin A 97% • Vitamin C 5% • Calcium 3% • Iron 71%

8.   Avocado smoothie

Avocado is a nutritional powerhouse rich in carotenoids, vitamin E, lutein, glutathione and oleic acid which fights off cancer. It is naturally high in dietary fibers and healthy fatty acids which are essential in colon cancer prevention.

Ingredients:

2 Avocadoes, pitted and sliced

1 cup Low-fat milk

1 Tbsp. Honey

5 Ice cubes

Preparation:

Throw in all ingredients in a blender. Blend well and enjoy.

Serving Size 265 g

Amount per Serving:

Calories 166

Calories from Fat 21

Total Fat 2.4g4%

Saturated Fat 1.5g

Cholesterol 12mg

Sodium 108mg

Potassium 377mg

Total Carbohydrates 29.5g

Sugars 29.9g

Protein 8.3g

Vitamin A 10% • Vitamin C 0%• Calcium 29% • Iron 1%

9.   Creamy macaroni and cheese

Studies show that milk and cheese protect against colon cancer. Calcium suppresses tumour cell proliferation, promotes terminal cell differentiation and induces apoptosis of colorectal tumour cells.

Ingredients:

1 cup Elbow macaroni, uncooked

1 1/2 Tbsp. Butter
1 ½ cups Cheddar cheese
2 Eggs, beaten

2 Tbsp. flour

½ cup Onion, minced

½ tsp. Paprika

½ tsp. Nutmeg

1/2 tsp. Salt

1 cup Low-fat milk

1/2 tsp. Dry mustard

1/2 teaspoon black pepper

Preparation:

Boil the macaroni in a saucepan for about 7 minutes or until macaroni is soft. Drain. In a medium saucepan, over low heat, melt butter and slowly stir in the milk. Add the cheese, stir until cheese melts. Add the eggs, mustard and onion then stir. Season with paprika, nutmeg, salt, and black pepper. Stir well then add drained macaroni. Gently stir until macaroni is completely covered in sauce. Serve and enjoy!

Serving Size 229 g

Amount per Serving:

Calories 492

Calories from Fat 261

Total Fat 29.0g

Saturated Fat 17.2g

Trans Fat 0.0g

Cholesterol 188mg

Sodium 859mg

Potassium 332mg

Total Carbohydrates 32.5g

Dietary Fiber 1.8g

Sugars 6.5g

Protein 25.2g

Vitamin A 25% • Vitamin C 3% • Calcium 54% • Iron 13%

10.   Blueberry yogurt

Studies show that yogurt is protective against colorectal cancer. The probiotic bacteria in yogurt prevents growth of pathogens. Its high dietary fiber accelerates bowel movement and promotes fast waste elimination. Yogurt is a good source of easily absorbable calcium and vitamin D both essential in colon cancer prevention.

Ingredients:

4 cups Blueberries

4 tbsp. Fresh lemon juice

1 cup Honey

1/4 tsp. Salt

1/4 tsp. Cinnamon

2 cups Low-fat plain yogurt

3/4 cup Whole milk

Preparation:

In a medium saucepan, over medium heat, combine blueberries, lemon juice, honey, salt and cinnamon. Stir until ingredients are well blended. Remove from heat. Transfer blueberry mixture into a large bowl. Mash the blueberries with a potato masher while heating. Cool for

10 minutes. Stir in the yogurt and milk, mix well until completely incorporated. Chill mixture in the refrigerator. Process blueberry yogurt mixture in ice cream maker for 30 minutes. Serve and enjoy.

Serving Size 414 g

Amount per Serving:

Calories 459

Calories from Fat 32

Total Fat 3.6g

Saturated Fat 2.2g

Trans Fat 0.0g

Cholesterol 12mg

Sodium 259mg

Potassium 527mg

Total Carbohydrates 102.0g

Dietary Fiber 3.8g

Sugars 95.3g

Protein 9.9g

Vitamin A 2% • Vitamin C 52% • Calcium 28% • Iron 14%

11. Chocolate cornflakes cake

Cereals contain fiber, vitamins, minerals and antioxidants. Consumption of cereals help ensure healthy digestive system and reduce the risk of bowel cancer.

Ingredients:

3 cups Cornflakes

3 Tbsp. Honey

100 g. Butter

150g. Cocoa powder

Preparation:

In a bowl, melt the chocolate, syrup and butter together using a microwave. Stir in the cornflakes. Spoon in one tablespoon of cornflakes mixture into 15 muffin liners. Refrigerate to set.

Serving Size 132 g

Amount per Serving:

Calories 514

Calories from Fat 302

Total Fat 33.6g

Saturated Fat 21.0g

Trans Fat 0.0g

Cholesterol 72mg

Sodium 402mg

Potassium 1318mg

Total Carbohydrates 68.7g

Dietary Fiber 15.9g

Sugars 21.1g

Protein 11.4g

Vitamin A 27% • Vitamin C 10% • Calcium 6% • Iron 89%

12.   Broccoli soup

Studies show that broccoli contain isothiocyanates, which are especially effective in fighting off several cancer cells of the lung, breast and colon. It appears to block and remove mutant genes associated with cancer growth.

Ingredients:

1/2 cup coconut oil

1 onion, chopped

2 cups Broccoli

½ cup Celery

4 cans (14.5) chicken broth

300 g. Cheddar cheese

2 cups milk

1 Tbsp. Garlic powder

2/3 cup Cornstarch

Preparation:

In a pot, pour coconut oil over medium heat. Cook onion in coconut oil until tender. Stir in broccoli and pour chicken broth. Simmer for 15 minutes or until broccoli is tender. Reduce heat and stir in cheese cubes, milk and garlic powder. Stir well. In a small bowl, dissolve cornstarch into 1 cup water. Pour cornstarch mixture into soup. Stir continuously until consistency is thick. Throw in celery and cook for 2 more minutes. Remove from heat and serve hot.

Serving Size 464 g

Amount per Serving:

Calories 389

Calories from Fat 243

Total Fat 27.0g

Saturated Fat 16.4g

Trans Fat 0.0g

Cholesterol 75mg

Sodium 1301mg

Potassium 451mg

Total Carbohydrates 18.1g

Dietary Fiber 1.2g5%

Sugars 5.1g

Protein 18.5g

Vitamin A 18% • Vitamin C 36% • Calcium 38% • Iron 7%

13.   Cod on creamed spinach

Spinach contains a high amount of beta-carotene that help fight colon cancer. A study done by Nutrition and Cancer show that people who ate cooked green vegetables, including spinach, once a day lowered the risk of colon cancer to 24 percent.

Ingredients:

2 fillet Cod

1 Tbsp. Olive oil

1 Tbsp Butter

1/4 cup Onion, chopped

1 Tbsp. Garlic, minced

1/2 cup Whipping cream

1/8 tsp Nutmeg

1 Tbsp. Dried thyme, ground

1/8 Salt

1/8 Pepper

Preparation:

Rub cod with thyme, salt and pepper. In a skillet, over medium heat, cook cod in olive oil for 7 minutes on each side or until light brown. Remove from heat and set aside.

Boil the spinach leaves in water over high heat for 5 minutes then drain. Pat leaves dry with a paper towel. Chop coarsely into shredded pieces. In a skillet, over medium-high heat, heat the butter and add the garlic and onion. Sauté until garlic is golden brown and onion is translucent. Pour the whipping cream and stir. Add nutmeg, salt and pepper and stir. Cook until mixture begins to boil and thicken. Throw in the drained spinach. Reduce heat to make consistency of cream thicker. Transfer to a plate with the cod. Serve immediately and enjoy.

Serving Size 129 g

Amount per Serving:

Calories 430

Calories from Fat 400

Total Fat 44.4g

Saturated Fat 21.0g

Cholesterol 97mg

Sodium 126mg

Potassium 160mg

Total Carbohydrates 9.1g

Dietary Fiber 1.9g

Sugars 1.5g

Protein 2.5g

Vitamin A 21% • Vitamin C 11% • Calcium 12% • Iron 20%

14.   Steamed fish and bok choy in oyster sauce

Bok choy is loaded with essential vitamins, nutrients and antioxidant. Cruciferous vegetables such as bok choy lowers the risk of colon cancer because of the glocosinolates it contain, that are converted into isothiocyanates, compounds that help the body fight cancer. Researchers estimate that eating lots of cruciferous vegetables could lower your risk of breast and colon cancer by 40 percent

Ingredients:

5 bunches Bok choy

2 Cream dory fillets

½ cup Oyster sauce

½ tsp. Ginger, minced

¼ tsp. Olive oil

1/4 tsp. Salt

1/4 tsp Pepper

Preparation:

In a small bowl, combine olive oil, ginger, salt and pepper. Rub fish with this mixture. Steam bok choy and fish for 30 minutes. Take out bok choy from steamer after 10 minutes. Transfer to a serving plate and drizzle with oyster sauce.

Serving Size 36 g

Amount per Serving:

Calories 3

1Calories from Fat 12

Total Fat 1.3g

Cholesterol 0mg

Sodium 1456mg

Potassium 36mg

Total Carbohydrates 4.5g

Protein 0.6g

Vitamin A 0% • Vitamin C 0% • Calcium 1% • Iron 2%

15.   Choco nutty apple smoothie

Studies show that apples may prevent colon cancer because of it strong antioxidant activity and flavonoids present in apple peels.

Ingredients:

3 Apples, chopped

1 cup Almond milk

1 Tbsp. Walnuts, ground

½ tsp. Cocoa powder

Preparation:

Throw in all ingredients in a blender. Blend well and enjoy!

Serving Size 274 g

Amount per Serving:

Calories 475

Calories from Fat 284

Total Fat 31.6g49%

Saturated Fat 25.5g

Trans Fat 0.0g

Cholesterol 0mg

Sodium 21mg

Potassium 705mg

Total Carbohydrates 53.5g

Dietary Fiber 11.1g4

Sugars 38.9g

Protein 4.7g

Vitamin A 0% • Vitamin C 48% • Calcium 2%   •   Iron 20%

16.   Stir fried watercress in garlic and onion

Consumption of garlic and onion significantly lower the risk of colon cancer. It also contains natural antibacterial, anti-viral, anti-fungal, and anti-inflammatory properties.

Ingredients:

100 g. Watercress

1 cup Shiitake mushroom

2 Tbsp. Garlic

2 Tbsp. Onion

1 Tbsp. Oyster sauce

1 Tbsp. Olive oil

1/8 tsp. Pepper

Preparation:

In a skillet, over medium-heat, sauté the garlic and onion in olive oil. Cook until garlic is light brown and onions are translucent. Add the oyster sauce, watercress and shiitake mushroom. Cover with a lid for 5 minutes. Remove the cover and garnish with pepper.

Serving Size 274 g

Amount per Serving:

Calories 475

Calories from Fat 284

Total Fat 31.6g49%

Saturated Fat 25.5g

Trans Fat 0.0g

Cholesterol 0mg

Sodium 21mg

Potassium 705mg

Total Carbohydrates 53.5g

Dietary Fiber 11.1g

Sugars 38.9g

Protein 4.7g

Vitamin A 0% • Vitamin C 48% • Calcium 2% •Iron 20%

17.   Turmeric curry chicken

The low occurrence of bowel cancer in India is associated with their diet rich in turmeric spices used in curry dishes. Its natural compound, curcumin, is a powerful antioxidant and anti-cancer agent. It inhibits the promotion/progression stages of carcinogenesis.

Ingredients:

400 g. Chicken, chopped in big chunks

2 cups Green papaya

5 cups Vegetable stock

1 Tbsp. Garlic

1 Tbsp. Onion

1 tsp. Turmeric powder

1/2 Tbsp. Curry powder

1 Tbsp. Ginger

1/8 tsp. Salt

1/8 tsp. Pepper

Preparation:

In a pot, over medium heat, sauté the garlic, onion and ginger. Cook garlic until light brown, onion is translucent and ginger is fragrant. Add chicken. Cook for 10 minutes until golden brown. Add vegetable stock, turmeric powder, curry powder and papaya. Stir then reduce heat and continue cooking for 5 minutes or until papaya is tender. Season with salt and pepper. Remove from heat and transfer to a serving bowl.

Serving Size 215 g

Amount per Serving:

Calories 329

Calories from Fat 59

Total Fat 6.6g

Saturated Fat 1.8g

Cholesterol 154mg

Sodium 276mg

Potassium 488mg

Total Carbohydrates 5.5g

Dietary Fiber 1.3g

Protein 58.8g

Vitamin A 1% • Vitamin C 4% • Calcium 5% • Iron 17%

18.   Strawberry banana smoothie

Flax seed is one of the best cancer-fighting foods. It is high in dietary fiber, omega 3 fat, and lignin. It actually contains the highest amount of lignan compared to any other food. Studies show that lignan reduces the size of cancerous tumors.

Ingredients:

4 cups Frozen strawberries

1 Banana

1 tsp. Flax seed

1 cup Low-fat plain vanilla yogurt

Preparation:

Throw in all ingredients in a blender. Blend well and enjoy!

Serving Size 363 g

Amount per Serving:

Calories 159

Calories from Fat 5

Total Fat 0.6g

Trans Fat 0.0g

Cholesterol 0mg

Sodium 1mg

Potassium 221mg

Total Carbohydrates 39.8g

Dietary Fiber 7.9g

Sugars 25.1g

Protein 0.9g

Vitamin A 1% • Vitamin C 189% • Calcium 4% • Iron 11%

19.   Almond quinoa with blueberries

Quinoa is an excellent source of fiber the colon needs. It is high in protein, minerals and essential amino acids.

Ingredients:

1 cup Quinoa, rinsed and soaked overnight

1/2 cup Almonds, slivered and blanched

1/2 cup Dried blueberries

1 tsp Olive oil

2 cups Vegetable stock

1/2 tsp Salt

1 Cinnamon stick

Preparation:

Rinse the soaked quinoa to remove its toxic saponin coating. Drain.

In a skillet, over medium heat, toast the sliced almonds in olive oil until golden brown. Remove from heat and set aside. Place the quinoa in the pan, stir and toast until dry. Add vegetable stock, salt, cinnamon stick and dried blueberries. Cover with a lid, bring to boil then simmer and cook for 10 minutes until all liquid is absorbed. Remove from heat and allow to sit while covered. Fluff gently using a fork and serve.

Serving Size 149 g

Amount per Serving:

Calories 491

Calories from Fat 175

Total Fat 19.5g

Saturated Fat 1.8g

Trans Fat 0.0g

Cholesterol 0mg

Sodium 586mg

Potassium 681mg

Total Carbohydrates 64.9g

Dietary Fiber 9.8g3

Sugars 4.6g

Protein 17.3g

Vitamin A 0%•Vitamin C 10%•Calcium 10%•Iron 29%

20.   Quick and easy avocado and tomato sandwich

Avocado is rich in cancer-fighting agent called carotenoids, present in the dark-green portion of the flesh that is closes to the skin.

Ingredients:

2 slices Whole-wheat bread

2 Tbsp. Avocado, mashed

1 small Tomato, thinly sliced

Preparation:

Spread the avocado on the two slices of bread, layer with tomatoes, cover with another slice of bread then enjoy!

Serving Size 165 g

Amount per Serving:

Calories 192

Calories from Fat 51

Total Fat 5.6g

Saturated Fat 1.2g

Trans Fat 0.5g

Cholesterol 0mg

Sodium 270mg

Potassium 443mg

Total Carbohydrates 28.2g

Dietary Fiber 6.1g

Sugars 5.6g

Protein 8.4g

Vitamin A 16% • Vitamin C 24% • Calcium 7% • Iron10%

21.   Mustard leaves kebab

Mustard leaves is packed with vitamins, minerals, essential amino acids and is rich in antioxidants. It reduces the risk of colon cancer and cancer in general because of the compound, glocosinolates which in turn produce isothiocyanates, which is a potent cancer-fighting metabolite.

Ingredients:

500g. Ground beef

1 cup Mustard leaves, minced

1 Tbsp. Onion

1/8 tsp. Dried pepper flakes

1/2 Tbsp. Coriander

1/2 Tbsp. Cumin

1 Tbsp. Butter

1/8 tsp. Olive oil

Salt and pepper to taste

Preparation:

Preheat the oven in 350F.

In a bowl, combine the meat, minced mustard leaves, onion, coriander, cumin, pepper flakes, salt and pepper. Knead the mixture with hands and form into four rectangle shaped kebabs. Cover the kebabs with olive oil using a brush. Grill in the oven for 15 minutes.

Serving Size 264 g

Amount per Serving:

Calories 526

Calories from Fat 198

Total Fat 22.0g

Saturated Fat 9.6g

Cholesterol 239mg

Sodium 208mg

Potassium 1045mg

Total Carbohydrates 1.2g

Protein 76.3g

Vitamin A 4% • Vitamin C 1% • Calcium 2% • Iron 267%

22. Chicken collard greens wrap

Consumption of collard greens especially reduces the risk of colon cancer. It contains four cancer-preventive properties which are derived from glucosinolates.

Ingredients:

4 Whole wheat tortilla wraps

200 g. Cooked chicken, strips

½ cup Collard greens, steamed

1/2 cup Cheddar cheese, grated

½ Tbsp. Onion

1 1/2 Tbsp. Light mayonnaise

1 tsp. Dijon mustard

1/8 tsp. Salt

1/8 tsp. Pepper

½ tsp. Sugar

Preparation:

In a bowl, combine all ingredients except for chicken then mix well. Spoon in the mixture and spread on the tortilla wrap. Layer with chicken strips and cheese on top. Roll the wrap and enjoy!

Serving Size 157 g

Amount per Serving:

Calories 318

Calories from Fat 146

Total Fat 16.2g

Saturated Fat 7.4g

Trans Fat 0.0g

Cholesterol 110mg

Sodium 495mg

Potassium 224mg

Total Carbohydrates 5.1g

Dietary Fiber 0.5g

Sugars 2.0g

Protein 36.5g

Vitamin A 14% • Vitamin C 6% • Calcium 23% • Iron 7%

23.   Steamed vegetables

Broccoli is the best vegetable that prevents disease and cancer. Raw broccoli contains diinodylmethane and sulforaphane which are the two most powerful anti-cancerous agents in nature. Lightly cooked broccoli is beneficial to the colon.

Ingredients:

2 cups Broccoli, halved

¾ cup Zucchini, thinly sliced

½ cup Red bell pepper thinly sliced

½ cup Carrots, thinly sliced

2 cups Water

1/8 tsp. Salt

1/8 tsp. Pepper

½ tsp. Garlic powder

1 tsp. Sesame oil

Preparation:

In a large ceramic, microwavable bowl, add the broccoli, zucchini, red bell pepper and carrots. Add water and drizzle with sesame oil. Cover tightly with a ceramic or stoneware plate. Microwave on high for 4 minutes. Carefully remove the cover then add salt and pepper.

Serving Size 268 g

Amount per Serving:

Calories 48

Calories from Fat 16

Total Fat 1.8g

Trans Fat 0.0g

Cholesterol 0mg

Sodium 137mg

Potassium 333mg

Total Carbohydrates 7.2g

Dietary Fiber 2.4g

Sugars 2.5g

Protein 2.3g

Vitamin A 70% • Vitamin C 100% • Calcium 4% • Iron 4%

24.   Grilled chicken

Colon cancer can be prevented by avoiding red meat. A healthy substitute is to consume the healthy white meat of chicken. Consumption of chicken has been found to actually reduce the risk of colorectal cancer.

Ingredients:

400 g. Chicken breast fillets

1 tsp. Fresh thyme

1 Tbsp. Garlic

½ tsp. Oregano

½ tsp. Freshly ground pepper

½ tsp. Kosher salt

6 Tbsp. Olive oil

Preparation:

In a Ziploc bag, combine all ingredients except for chicken, mix well. Add the chicken in the Ziploc bag then refrigerate for at least 1 hour. Set electric grill to 350F. Grease the grill with olive oil. Place the chicken on the grill. Grill for 8 to 12 minutes on each side. Transfer to a serving plate and enjoy!

Serving Size 168 g

Amount per Serving:

Calories 500

Calories from Fat 342

Total Fat 38.0g58%

Saturated Fat 6.7g

Cholesterol 119mg

Sodium 503mg

Potassium 347mg

Total Carbohydrates 1.5g

Protein 38.9g

Vitamin A 2% • Vitamin C 2% • Calcium 4% • Iron 13%

25.   Garlic mushroom taco salad

Studies show that mushrooms contain numerous compound with anti-cancer properties such as lectins, lentinan and various β-glucans. Mushrooms contain anti-inflammatory, antivarl, cholesterol-reducing and immune enhance properties as well.

Ingredients:

¾ cup Crimini mushroom, minced

6 cups Lettuce, shredded

1 Avocado, chopped

3 Tbsp. Onion

3 Tbsp. Garlic

1 Tbsp. Olive oil

1 cup Lean ground beef

½ cup Red pepper, chopped

1/2 tsp. Dried thyme leaves

1/2 tsp. dried Oregano leaves

1/2 tsp. Ground mustard

2 Tbsp. Tomato paste

1 can Diced tomatoes

1/2 cup Cheddar cheese, shredded

1/4 cup Fresh cilantro, chopped

Preparation:

Process the onion, garlic and mushroom in a food processor. Blend well until finely chopped. In a large non-stick skillet, over medium-heat, heat the oil and sauté the ground beef for 5 minutes or until brown. Add the mushroom mixture, oregano, thyme, mustard and red pepper. Cook for 5 minutes or until tender. Add the tomatoes and tomato paste. Simmer until thick or for about 10 minutes. Divide the lettuce evenly between four plates. Top with meat mixture, cheese, avocado and cilantro.

Serving Size 267 g

Amount per Serving:

Calories 308

Calories from Fat 221

Total Fat 24.6g

Saturated Fat 7.4g

Trans Fat 0.0g

Cholesterol 20mg

Sodium 142mg

Potassium 789mg

Total Carbohydrates 17.8g

Dietary Fiber 6.7g

Sugars 4.7g

Protein 8.4g

Vitamin A 25% • Vitamin C 94% • Calcium 18% • Iron 25%

26.   Chicken salad sandwich on a whole-grain bread

Studies show that people who consume chicken several times a week decrease the risk of developing precancerous polyps in the colon and the occurrence of malignant tumors.

Ingredients:

4 slices Whole wheat bread

2 Cooked boneless chicken breasts, shredded

1 stalk celery

2 Tbsp. Onion

1 cup Celery, chopped

1 1/2 cup Mayonnaise

2 Tbsp. Fresh lemon juice

1/8 tsp. Salt

1/8 tsp. Pepper

1 Tbsp. Fresh parsley

1 Tbsp. Dill

Preparation:

In a medium size bowl, mix all ingredients. Scoop a

tablespoon or two on a slice of bread, cover with another slice and enjoy!

Serving Size 144 g

Amount per Serving:

Calories 160

Calories from Fat 20

Total Fat 2.2g

Saturated Fat 0.6g

Trans Fat 0.5g

Cholesterol 0mg

Sodium 467mg

Potassium 389mg

Total Carbohydrates 27.2g

Dietary Fiber 5.3g

Sugars 4.7g

Protein 8.3g

Vitamin A 10% • Vitamin C 21% • Calcium 12% • Iron 13%

27.   Baked cod over sweet potatoes, carrots and peas

Codfish is a good source of essential vitamins and minerals such as vitamin B-6, vitamin B-12, vitamin D, phosphorous, potassium and selenium. Studies show that cod fish can prevent colon cancer by inhibiting metastasis of cancer cell due to the high content of omega-6 fatty acid present in the fish.

Ingredients:

4 fillet Cod

1 Tbsp. Olive oil

1 Tbsp. Onion, chopped

1 Tbsp. Garlic, minced

1/2 cup Black olives, pitted

3/4 cup White wine

3/4 cup Cherry tomatoes, quartered

1 lemon, zested and juiced

2 large Potatoes, peeled and chopped

1 cup Carrots, roundly and thinly sliced

1/4 cup Peas

1/4 cup Fresh basil leaves

Preparation:

Preheat oven to 400F.

In a small skillet, sauté garlic and onion in olive oil until garlic is light brown and onion is translucent. Add the tomato, carrots and peas and basil leaves. Stir and lower heat. Simmer for 10 minutes. Place cod in a large baking dish. Add wine and olives. Add the cooked garlic, onion, tomatoes, carrots and peas around the cod. Add the lemon juice and zest. Season with parsley, salt and pepper. Bake in the oven for 20 minutes or until fish is flaky. Serve and enjoy!

Serving Size 434 g

Amount per Serving:

Calories 323

Calories from Fat 67

Total Fat 7.5g11%

Saturated Fat 1.1g

Trans Fat 0.0g

Cholesterol 0mg

Sodium 242mg

Potassium 1337mg

Total Carbohydrates 50.0g

Dietary Fiber 8.8g

Sugars 7.1g

Protein 6.0g

Vitamin A 136% • Vitamin C 105% • Calcium 8% • Iron 15%

28. Fried spring rolls with moringa oleifera

Moringa oleifera is also called as "miracle tree" because almost all of its part from the root to its leaves have anticancer, hepatoprotective, hypoglycemic, anti-inflammatory, antibacterial, antifungal, antiviral, and antisickling effects.

Ingredients:

500 g. Ground pork

½ cup Green onions

1 cup Carrots, minced

1/2 cup Onion, minced

2 Eggs

1 ½ tsp. Salt

2 tsp. Garlic powder

¼ cup Parsley, minced

1 cup Moringa oleifera leaves, minced

30 pcs. Spring roll wrapper

4 cups cococut oil

Preparation:

In a mixing bowl, combine all ingredients. Mix well. Scoop a 1 ½ tbsp. of the pork mixture in a spring roll wrapper and wrap. Heat the cooking oil in a deep fryer. Deep fry the spring roll for 10-12 minutes or until golden brown. Remove from oil and remove excess oil by placing on top of a serving platter lined with napkin. Share and enjoy!

Serving Size 122 g

Amount per Serving:

Calories 619

Calories from Fat 578

Total Fat 64.2g

Saturated Fat 12.8g

Trans Fat 0.0g

Cholesterol 49mg

Sodium 284mg

Potassium 211mg

Total Carbohydrates 1.9g

Sugars 0.8g

Protein 10.4g

Vitamin A 29% • Vitamin C 5% • Calcium 1% • Iron 4%

29.   Tomato smoothie

Tomatoes contain a natural antioxidant, lycopene, which reduces the chance of colorectal and stomach cancer. It is also rich in beta-carotene, vitamin A and vitamin C.

Ingredients:

6 medium Tomatoes, quartered

1 cup Carrots, chopped

1 stalk Celery, chopped

2 Tbsp. Fresh lemon juice

2 Tbsp. Honey

Preparation:

Freeze chopped tomatoes and carrots for one hour. Toss in all ingredients in a blender and blend well. Pour into a long stemmed glass and enjoy chilled!

Serving Size 313 g

Amount per Serving:

Calories 105

Calories from Fat 5

Total Fat 0.6g

Trans Fat 0.0g

Cholesterol 0mg

Sodium 44mg

Potassium 735mg

Total Carbohydrates 25.1g

Dietary Fiber 4.0g1

Sugars 20.1g

Protein 2.6g

Vitamin A 164% • Vitamin C 68% • Calcium 4% • Iron 5%

30.   Mixed berry custard pie

Berries are effective in preventing occurrence of colon cancer because it contains powerful antioxidants that triggers apoptosis among cancerous cells.

Ingredients:

1 cup Blueberries

½ cup Raspberries

4 large eggs

3/4 cup Low-fat milk

1 tsp. Vanilla extract

1/2 cup Sugar

1 9-inch Store-bought unbaked pie crust

Preparation:

Preheat oven to 350F.

In a medium bowl, combine egg, sugar, milk and vanilla. Beat well. Cover bottom of the pie crust with the berries. Pour the egg mixture on top. Bake until center is set or about 40-45 minutes. Remove from the oven and cool to room temperature. Serve and enjoy!

Serving Size 231 g

Amount per Serving:

Calories 288

Calories from Fat 68

Total Fat 7.5g

Saturated Fat 2.5g

Cholesterol 251mg

Sodium 121mg

Potassium 251mg

Total Carbohydrates 46.5g

Dietary Fiber 2.5g

Sugars 42.9g

Protein 11.1g

Vitamin A 9% • Vitamin C 22% •Calcium 11% • Iron 11%

31. Chicken stir fry with mixed peppers

Bell peppers especially red bell pepper contain plenty of carotenoids, lycopene and beta-carotene which help reduce the risk of colon cancer and growth of polyps cells. It is also a good source of N-acetylcysteine (NAC), a natural compound which has an anti-cancer property.

Ingredients:

2 Boneless skinless chicken breasts, cut into strips

1 Red bell pepper, ribs and seeds removed, chopped into strips

1 Yellow pepper, ribs and seeds removed, chopped into strips

1 Green pepper, ribs and seeds removed, chopped into strips

2 tsp. Ginger, minced

1 Tbsp. Garlic, minced

1 Tbsp. Onion, minced

1 Tbsp. Fish sauce

2 Tbsp. Olive oil

½ tsp. Sesame oil

Preparation:

In a medium skillet, sauté the onion and garlic in olive oil until onion is translucent and garlic is light brown. Stir fry the chicken until thoroughly cook or for until 3 to 4 minutes. Add the peppers, ginger, and fish sauce.

Serving Size 239 g

Amount per Serving:

Calories 204

Calories from Fat 141

Total Fat 15.7g

Saturated Fat 2.2g

Cholesterol 0mg

Sodium 701mg

Potassium 488mg

Total Carbohydrates 16.6g

Dietary Fiber 3.1g

Sugars 5.1g

Protein 3.0g

Vitamin A 48%•Vitamin C 559% • Calcium 4% • Iron 7%

32.   Carrot ginger turmeric smoothie

Turmeric and ginger are reportedly known to decrease the risk of colon polyps formation because of its main ingredient, curcumin, which is a powerful antioxidant.

Ingredients:

2 cups Carrots

1 large Banana

½ Tbsp. Ginger

¼ tsp. Turmeric, ground

1 cup Almond milk

3 Ice cubes

Preparation:

Combine all ingredients in a blender and blend well. Serve chilled.

Serving Size 300 g

Amount per Serving:

Calories 387

Calories from Fat 260

Total Fat 28.9g

Saturated Fat 25.5g

Trans Fat 0.0g

Cholesterol 0mg

Sodium 95mg

Potassium 936mg

Total Carbohydrates 34.1g

Dietary Fiber 7.3g

Sugars 17.8g

Protein 4.5g

Vitamin A 368% • Vitamin C 27% • Calcium 6% • Iron 15%

ADDITIONAL TITLES FROM THIS AUTHOR

70 Effective Meal Recipes to Prevent and Solve Being Overweight: Burn Fat Fast by Using Proper Dieting and Smart Nutrition

By

Joe Correa CSN

48 Acne Solving Meal Recipes: The Fast and Natural Path to Fixing Your Acne Problems in Less Than 10 Days!

By

Joe Correa CSN

41 Alzheimer's Preventing Meal Recipes: Reduce or Eliminate Your Alzheimer's Condition in 30 Days or Less!

By

Joe Correa CSN

70 Effective Breast Cancer Meal Recipes: Prevent and Fight Breast Cancer with Smart Nutrition and Powerful Foods

By

Joe Correa CSN

www.ingramcontent.com/pod-product-compliance
Lightning Source LLC
Chambersburg PA
CBHW030251030426
42336CB00009B/335